The Sweet Trap

Understanding The Role of Corn Syrups in The Obesity Epidemic

Table Of Content

Table Of Content

INTRODUCTION

The World Health Organization (WHO) describes obesity as a condition in which a person has a body mass index (BMI) of 30 kg/m2 or more. The availability and affordability of high-calorie, low-nutrient foods have facilitated a shift towards sedentary lifestyles, which is why this trend is most prominent in developed nations. Many health issues, such as an elevated risk of heart disease, stroke, diabetes, and several types of cancer, are linked to obesity. With the considerable negative effects of obesity on both the health of an individual and the health of society as a whole, there is increased interest in figuring out the root causes of the epidemic and creating measures for its effective prevention and treatment. One area of particular interest in this research is the role of dietary variables, notably the use of high quantities of added sugars, like corn syrup.

In the modern diet, especially in the United States, corn syrup is frequently used as a sweetener.

A Thorough overview of how corn syrup functions in the current diet and how it could affect obesity and other related health problems. The science of how corn syrup is processed by the body will be examined in the book, as well as the processes by which it might promote the onset of obesity and other related health problems. The book hopes to teach readers about the possible dangers of ingesting large amounts of corn syrup and other added sugars as well as practical advice on how to cut back on their use. Health experts, nutritionists, policymakers, and members of the general public who are interested in understanding the connection between diet and obesity will all find the book to be interesting. It will present a fair-minded and fact-based viewpoint on the function of corn syrup in the contemporary diet and practical guidance on how to choose healthier foods.

CHAPTER **1**

WHAT IS CORN SYRUP

Corn Syrup is a sweetener made from corn starch after processing it to change some of the glucose molecules into fructose molecules. The resulting syrup is a transparent, viscous liquid that is frequently added to processed meals, drinks, and baked goods. There are various kinds of Corn Syrup available, each with a unique glucose-to-fructose ratio. High fructose corn syrup (HFCS), the most popular variety used in the food sector, typically includes 42% to 55% fructose with the remainder being made up of glucose and other sugars. Because of its low cost, useful qualities, and capacity to improve the texture and shelf life of processed foods, corn syrup is frequently employed in the food business. It is frequently present in a variety of foods, including sodas, candies, cereal, baked goods, and even savory ones like ketchup and salad dressings.

The potential negative consequences of ingesting corn syrup, especially high fructose corn syrup, on one's health have been hotly contested. Its use has been linked by some researchers to the emergence of obesity, type 2 diabetes, and other health problems. As a result, attempts to minimize the consumption of corn syrup and other added sugars are ongoing.

<u>Types of corn Syrup and their production Processes</u>

There are various kinds of corn syrup, and each one has a different amount of fructose and glucose. Following are a few popular varieties of maize syrup:

1)Light corn syrup: This contains a larger amount of glucose and a lower proportion of fructose than regular corn syrup. To stop sugar crystals from forming, it is frequently used in baking and candy-making.

2)Dark corn syrup: Compared to light corn syrup, this variety of corn syrup contains a higher percentage of fructose and glucose.

It is frequently used in dishes that call for a stronger flavor, like gingerbread.

3)High Fructose Corn Syrup: Adding enzymes to corn starch causes some of the glucose to be converted into fructose, making high-fructose corn syrup (HFCS) a sweeter syrup. Processed foods and beverages frequently employ HFCS as a sweetener.

The process of making corn syrup includes the following steps:

1)Corn Milling: corn kernels are cleaned and milled to produce corn starch.

2)Starch hydrolysis: Enzymes are added to break down corn starch into glucose molecules.

3)Purification of glucose: Any contaminants or residual enzymes are taken out of the glucose syrup that is produced.

4)Fructose conversion: Other enzymes convert certain glucose molecules into fructose during the manufacturing of high fructose corn syrup.

5)Final Refining: The syrup is further processed to get rid of any impurities or off-flavors that could still be present.

The resulting corn syrup can be used as an ingredient in several food and beverages. While. Corn syrup is a common ingredient in many processed foods. It is important to use it sparingly as part of a balanced diet because excessive consumption of added sugars, such as corn syrup, can lead to health problems like obesity, type 2 diabetes, and other conditions that are related to these two.

<u>Common uses of Corn Syrup in the Food Industry</u>

Due to its useful qualities and sweetness, corn syrup is a frequent ingredient in the food business. Following are a few of the most typical applications for corn syrup:

1)Sweetener: In the food sector, corn syrup is a preferred sweetener. It is frequently used in a variety of culinary products, such as baked goods, candies, and soft drinks, as an alternative to sugar or other sweeteners.

2)Corn syrup can also be used to improve the texture of food products: Its viscosity and texture can enable goods like ice cream, sorbets, and other frozen sweets to have a better mouthfeel and texture.

3)Preservative: Certain food products may also contain corn syrup as a preservative. By impeding the growth of bacteria and other microbes that can contaminate food.

4)Binder: Corn syrup can serve as a binder in culinary products, holding ingredients together. Granola bars, cereal bars, and other snack foods frequently contain them.

5)Flavor Enhancer: Corn syrup is a taste enhancer that some dishes might benefit from. Its sweetness can assist in bringing other flavors in goods like ketchup, barbeque sauce, and other condiments into harmony.

6)Humectant: Corn syrup can operate as a humectant, which means it can aid food products to retain moisture. To keep baked goods like cookies and cakes wet and fresh for longer, it is frequently used in baking.

Overall, due to its functional qualities and capacity to improve the flavor, texture, and appearance of food products, corn syrup is a versatile ingredient that is frequently utilized in the food industry.

The nutritional Properties of corn syrup

Glucose, a simple sugar, is the main component of corn syrup. The following are a few of the main nutritional properties of corn syrup:

a)Calories: Corn Syrup is a high-calorie Sweetener. In 1/4 cup (60 mL) serving, there are roughly 240 calories.

b)Carbohydrates: The majority of Corn Syrup is made up of these fuel-producing molecules. In 1/4 cup (60 mL) serving, there are roughly 60 grams of carbs.

c)Sugar: Corn syrup is a source of sugar, which, if ingested in excess, can increase the risk of conditions like obesity and type 2 diabetes.

d)Fat: Corn syrup is entirely fat-free.

e)Protein: Corn syrup is essentially devoid of protein.

f)Minerals and vitamins: Corn syrup is not a very good source of minerals or vitamins.

It is important to note that in processed meals that are high in calories, sugar, and fat but poor in essential nutrients, Corn Syrup is frequently added. Overeating these items can lead to a poor diet and a higher risk of developing conditions like obesity and heart disease. So, as part of a balanced diet, it is advised to eat corn syrup and other sweeteners in moderation.

The Digestion of Corn Syrup

As earlier stated, Corn Syrup is a Sweetener derived from Corn Starch. It is produced via the addition of enzymes like alpha-amylase and glucoamylase that convert the starch in corn kernels into glucose. This procedure results in a syrup with a high concentration of glucose, a simple sugar that is simple to digest for the body. The process of breaking down corn syrup into smaller sugars like glucose and maltose starts in the mouth where the salivary enzyme amylase breaks down the syrup's carbs. The small intestine then allows these carbohydrates to enter the circulation. Glucose is carried by the bloodstream to the body's cells, where it is used as a fuel source. By instructing cells to absorb glucose from the blood, the pancreatic hormone insulin helps to control the amount of glucose in the bloodstream. If the body does not immediately require glucose for energy, it can be stored as glycogen in the muscles and liver for later use. But, if there is too much glucose, it can be turned into fat and stored as long-term energy in adipose tissue.

<u>NOTA BENE:</u>

Generally, corn syrup digests and is metabolized similarly to other simple sugars. However, drinking too much corn syrup can result in health issues like obesity, type 2 diabetes, and heart disease.

<u>The impact of Corn Syrup in the Body</u>

Like other sweets, the effects of corn syrup on the body vary depending on how much is ingested and how healthy the person is generally. The body can be impacted by corn syrup in the following ways:

1)blood sugar level spike: Because corn syrup contains a lot of glucose, blood sugar levels may rise quickly. For those who have diabetes, this might be challenging since their bodies might not be able to create enough insulin to control blood sugar levels.

2)Obesity and Weight Gain: Eating too much corn syrup and other sweets can cause weight gain and obesity. This is because artificial sweeteners increase calorie intake without offering many nutritional benefits.

3)Elevated risk of heart disease: According to studies. This may be because drinking large amounts of corn syrup might result in increased blood levels of triglycerides, a kind of fat linked to cardiovascular disease.

4)Dental issues: Eating sweet foods and beverages, such as corn syrup, can aggravate dental issues like tooth decay.

5)Addiction and desires: Some people may develop cravings for sugary foods and become hooked to the sweet flavor of corn syrup.

NOTA BENE:

Thus, even while corn syrup can be safely ingested in moderation, consuming too much of it might have harmful health effects.

Limit your intake of sugary meals and beverages and concentrate on eating a balanced diet with lots of healthy foods, fruits, and vegetables.

The Sweet Trap

CHAPTER **2**

THE MECHANISM RELATIONSHIP BETWEEN CORN SYRUP AND OBESITY.

Sweeteners like corn syrup are frequently found in processed meals and beverages including soda, baked goods, and candy. It yields either a mixture of glucose and fructose or a high concentration of glucose (in the form of corn syrup) (in the form of high-fructose corn syrup, or HFCS) Because it is a source of empty calories that might cause weight gain, some studies have suggested that eating large amounts of HFCS may lead to obesity. In other studies, HFCS consumption has also been associated with a higher risk of metabolic diseases such as type 2 diabetes and heart disease.

It's also important to remember that there is no single cause for obesity, which is a complicated disorder influenced by a variety of factors, including genetics, lifestyle, and environmental influences.

It is advised to eat a varied diet high in nutrient-dense foods while avoiding highly processed foods and added sugars is good for overall health and may help reduce the risk of obesity.

How Corn Syrup Spikes Blood Sugar Levels

Glucose, a form of sugar that quickly raises blood sugar levels when taken, is present in large amounts in corn syrup. Consuming corn syrup causes the sugars to break down into glucose, which is then taken into the bloodstream. When blood sugar levels rise, the body releases the hormone insulin, which tells cells to take up glucose from the blood and helps control blood sugar levels. Consuming corn syrup can be harmful to persons with diabetes or other diseases that impact how blood sugar is regulated. Consuming too much corn syrup can result in hyperglycemia,

or high blood sugar levels if the body is unable to create enough insulin to control blood sugar levels.

Repeated blood sugar increases have been linked to the emergence of type 2 diabetes as well as other health issues like kidney and heart disease over time.

NOTA BENE

Those with diabetes or other diseases that alter blood sugar levels should keep an eye on how much corn syrup and other sweeteners they consume. Along with developing a nutrition strategy that supports healthy blood sugar management, they should work closely with their doctor to ensure general health.

Corn Syrup and Insulin Resistance

Some evidence points to a connection between excessive corn syrup consumption and insulin resistance, which is a risk factor for type 2 diabetes.

High-fructose corn syrup (HFCS), sometimes known as corn syrup, is a sweetener that is frequently used in the production of processed foods and beverages.

It is made from Corn starch, and some of the glucose molecules are chemically changed into fructose during processing. The body's cells become less receptive to the hormone insulin, which is in charge of controlling blood sugar levels, as a result of a high intake of fructose, according to studies. Insulin resistance is a condition in which this happens. As a result of the body producing more insulin to counteract cells that have become resistant to it, type 2 diabetes and high blood sugar levels may eventually result.

One study indicated that rats on a high-fructose diet for six weeks exhibited evidence of insulin resistance as well as higher blood levels of triglycerides, a form of fat. This study was published in the Journal of Nutrition. Another study indicated that males who ingested large amounts of fructose had reduced insulin sensitivity and increased levels of inflammation in their bodies. This study was also published in the American Journal of Clinical Nutrition. It is important to note that although these studies point to a connection between corn syrup and insulin resistance, additional study is necessary to completely comprehend the processes underlying this association and to establish the safe intake levels for corn syrup.

The Impact of Corn Syrup on Metabolic Syndrome

The risk of type 2 diabetes, heart disease, and stroke is increased by a group of diseases known as metabolic syndrome. High blood pressure, high blood sugar, extra belly fat, and abnormal cholesterol or triglyceride levels are some of these problems.

High intakes of added sugars, especially corn syrup, have been linked in some studies to the development of metabolic syndrome.

The consequences of excessive sugar consumption and insulin resistance are one possible pathway. High blood sugar spikes are a result of insulin resistance, which happens when the body's cells stop responding to the actions of insulin.

Also, ingesting a lot of added sugars may cause you to have too much belly fat, which is an obvious defect of metabolic syndrome. This is due to the fact that excessive sugar consumption will result in a higher calorie intake, which is then deposited as belly fat. The metabolic syndrome may also be exacerbated by consuming large amounts of fructose, which is present in both high-fructose corn syrup and table sugar. This is because fructose is processed differently than glucose and may lead to an increase in insulin resistance and hepatic fat deposition.

NOTA BENE

The risk of developing metabolic syndrome and other linked chronic health disorders, however, can be decreased by restricting the use of processed foods and beverages that include added sugars, such as corn syrup.

The Addictive Properties of Corn Syrup and its Effect on Food Craving

Like other added sugars, corn syrup has addictive qualities that lead to food cravings and overeating. Dopamine, a neurotransmitter associated with pleasure and reward, is released by eating sugar, activating reward areas in the brain. Similar to the cycle of craving and reward-seeking behavior seen with addictive substances like narcotics, this can result in.

Furthermore, taking a lot of added sugars, like corn syrup, can cause your blood sugar levels to increase quickly followed by a crash, which can make you hungry and make you need more sugar. This cycle results in a pattern of overeating and supports the emergence of obesity as well as other health issues.

Also, people looking for a quick and fulfilling source of energy may find processed foods and beverages with added sugars—including corn syrup—attractive due to their widespread availability and low price.

This makes it more challenging to stop the loop of sugar cravings and addiction and can contribute to a tendency of overconsumption.

Overall, corn syrup's and other added sugars' addictive qualities can lead to food cravings and overeating, both of which can be harmful to one's health. Consuming fewer processed foods and drinks that include added sugars, such as corn syrup, may assist to end the cycle of sugar addiction and enhance general health.

CHAPTER **3**

THE FOOD INDUSTRY AND CORN SYRUP

The History of Corn Syrup in the Food Industry.

As a less costly alternative to cane sugar, corn syrup was initially created in the late 19th century. The starch in corn must be converted into glucose, a simple sugar that can be used as a sweetener, to make corn syrup. Early on, the creation of confectionery and baked products was the main usage of corn syrup.

The invention of high-fructose corn syrup (HFCS) at the turn of the 20th century increased the usage of corn syrup in the food industry. Adding enzymes to corn syrup causes some of the glucose to be converted into fructose, which is sweeter than glucose, and this process creates HFCS. Soft drinks, baked goods, and other processed foods frequently include HFCS. Due to their low cost and wide availability, corn syrup and HFCS have seen an increase in use in the food sector. Corn is a major crop in the United States, and the development of industrial-scale processing techniques has allowed for the production of enormous amounts of corn syrup and HFCS at comparatively low costs. Corn is a significant crop in the United States.

Alternatives to Corn Syrup

In the food sector, several alternatives to corn syrup are frequently utilized. These are a few instances:

1)**Honey:** Honey, a natural sweetener, is often used in baking and cooking. It's crucial to remember that honey still counts as added sugar and should only be consumed in moderation.

2)**Sugar Maples:** Another natural sweetener frequently used as a corn syrup replacement is maple syrup.

It has a distinctive flavor and can be cooked, baked, or used as a pancake and waffle topping.

3)Nectar from Agave: A natural sweetener made from the agave plant is called agave nectar. It can be replaced for corn syrup in many recipes because of its comparable consistency.

4)Brown rice syrup: Made from brown rice, brown rice syrup is a natural sweetener. It can be used in baking and cooking and has a moderate flavor.

5)Fruit juice concentrates: Apple or grape juice concentrate, for example, can be used as a natural sweetener in a variety of dishes. They can also give baked items more taste and moisture.

6)Stevia: The leaves of the Stevia rebaudiana plant are used to make Stevia, a natural sweetener. It can be substituted for sugar in many recipes because it is significantly sweeter. Stevia can, however, have a harsh aftertaste and may not be appropriate for all recipes, so it is crucial to keep that in mind.

<u>NOTA BENE</u>

Overall, there are several corn syrup substitutes that are acceptable for usage in the food industry. While selecting a replacement, it's crucial to keep things like flavor, consistency, and accessibility in mind. Also, it's critical to remember that all sweeteners should be used moderately as part of a healthy diet.

<u>Natural sweeteners: advantages and disadvantages</u>

Sweetening substances known as natural sweeteners come from organic sources like plants, fruits, and honey. They each have advantages and disadvantages while being frequently regarded as better alternatives to high fructose corn syrup and artificial sweeteners.

These are some instances of natural sweeteners along with their advantages and disadvantages:

1)Honey: Bees generate the natural sweetener known as honey. It possesses anti-inflammatory qualities and antioxidants. Unfortunately, honey contains a lot of calories and raises blood sugar levels.

2)Maple syrup: Made from the sap of maple trees, maple syrup is a natural sweetener. Minerals like calcium and potassium are present. It should be consumed in moderation nevertheless because it is heavy in calories.

3)Agave nectar: Made from the agave plant, agave nectar is a natural sweetener. It doesn't induce a sharp rise in blood sugar levels because it has a lower glycemic index than table sugar. Due to its high fructose content, it should only be consumed occasionally.

4)Stevia: The leaves of the Stevia rebaudiana plant are used to make Stevia, a natural sweetener. It contains no calories and is far sweeter than sugar. Stevia, however, might leave some people with a bitter aftertaste.

5)Fruit juice concentrates: Fruit juice concentrates are naturally occurring sugars that come from fruits, such as apple or grape juice concentrate. They can enhance the flavor and moisture of baked goods and contain vitamins and minerals. They should only be used in moderation though because they are also abundant in natural sugars.

NOTA BENE

In general, natural sweeteners can be a better option than high fructose corn syrup and artificial sweeteners. Nonetheless, as part of a balanced diet, it is crucial to utilize them in moderation. When selecting a natural sweetener, it's crucial to keep things like flavor, texture, and availability in mind.

The Importance of Government Regulation on Alternative Sweeteners and Corn Syrup.

To guarantee that they are safe for consumption and that their labels are accurate, the government has a responsibility to play in regulating corn syrup and other sweeteners. The following are some methods by which the government controls sweeteners:

1)Labeling specifications: The government mandates that food producers list each component on the product's packaging. Sweeteners are included, and the labeling needs to be precise and understandable. For how items can be marketed and branded as "natural" or "organic," the FDA has certain regulations.

2)Safety requirements: The government establishes safety requirements for sweeteners, including the maximum permissible concentrations of particular components. For instance, the FDA places restrictions on the maximum amount of lead that can be found in sweeteners like honey and maple syrup.

3)Before they may be utilized in food items, some sweeteners must go through an approval process: For instance, the FDA must approve high-intensity sweeteners like stevia and monk fruit before they may be used in foods and beverages.

4)Import restrictions: If a country's sweeteners don't meet safety requirements, the government may limit their importation. For instance, if it is discovered that honey from a particular country has dangerous chemicals or pollutants, the FDA may decide to ban its importation.

Generally, the government has a significant impact on the regulation of sweeteners to guarantee their safety and correct labeling. This supports consumer safety and increases accountability in the food sector. Government restrictions regarding sweeteners are expected to change as worries about the health implications of sugar and corn syrup continue to rise.

healthier diets can have a positive impact on overall health and well-being. Here are some recommendations:

Read food labels: Corn syrup is often hidden in processed foods, so it is important to read the labels of all packaged foods before consuming them. Look for foods that do not contain corn syrup or other added sugars.

1)Cook at home: Cooking at home can help you control the ingredients and the amount of sugar in your meals. Always for natural sweeteners like honey or maple syrup instead of corn syrup.

2)Choose whole foods: Whole foods like fruits, vegetables, whole grains, and lean protein sources are naturally low in added sugars and high in nutrients. Incorporate them into your meals and snacks as much as possible.

3)Limit sugary beverages: Soda, fruit juices, and other sugary drinks are often high in corn syrup and can contribute to excessive sugar consumption. Choose water, unsweetened tea or coffee, or sparkling water instead.

4)Be mindful of portion sizes: Even natural sweeteners like honey and maple syrup should be consumed in moderation. Pay attention to portion sizes and limit added sugars to no more than 10% of your daily caloric intake.

5)Get support: Making dietary changes can be challenging, but having support can make it easier. Consider working with a registered dietitian or joining a support group to help you achieve your health goals.

CONCLUSION

There is still much work to be done to address the obesity epidemic and promote healthier diets. It will take a concerted effort from individuals, governments, and the food industry to make significant progress. The future of corn syrup and the obesity epidemic is uncertain, but there are promising signs of progress toward healthier diets and lifestyles. By continuing to raise awareness, promote healthy choices, and support policies and initiatives that promote public health, we can work towards a future where obesity and related health problems are no longer major public health concerns.